THE SCOPE OF PRACTICE

for

ACADEMIC NURSE EDUCATORS

&

ACADEMIC CLINICAL NURSE EDUCATORS

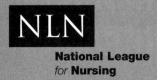

National League
for **Nursing**

THE SCOPE OF PRACTICE

for
ACADEMIC NURSE EDUCATORS

&

ACADEMIC CLINICAL NURSE EDUCATORS

Third Edition

Edited by:

Linda S. Christensen, EdD, JD, RN, CNE

Larry E. Simmons, PhD, RN, CNE, NEA-BC

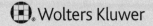

Philadelphia • Baltimore • New York • London
Buenos Aires • Hong Kong • Sydney • Tokyo

Vice President and Publisher: Julie K. Stegman
Director of Nursing Content Publishing: Renee Gagliardi
Director of Product Development: Jennifer K. Forestieri
Senior Development Editor: Meredith L. Brittain
Marketing Manager: Brittany Clements
Editorial Assistant: Molly Kennedy
Design Coordinator: Terry Mallon
Senior Production Project Manager: Alicia Jackson
Manufacturing Coordinator: Karin Duffield
Prepress Vendor: Aptara, Inc.

Christensen, L. S., and Simmons, L. E. (2020). *The Scope of Practice for Academic Nurse Educators and Academic Clinical Nurse Educators* (3rd ed.). Washington, DC: National League for Nursing.

9 8 7 6 5 4 3 2 1

Printed in USA

Library of Congress Cataloging-in-Publication Data

ISBN-13: 978-1-97515-192-8
Library of Congress Control Number: 2019917030
Cataloging in Publication data available on request from publisher.

---

shop.lww.com   www.NLN.org

DRC1119

About the Editors

Linda S. Christensen, EdD, JD, RN, CNE is Chief Governance Officer for the National League for Nursing and has been with the National League for Nursing for the past 10 years. Her work at the National League for Nursing has included administrative oversight of the Academic Nurse Educator Certification Program, where she has assisted with program administration and new certification program development. She has over 35 years of experience in nursing education, with expertise in nursing education administration, nursing program development, curriculum development, and 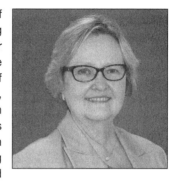 evaluation. She has taught both graduate and undergraduate nursing, both on campus and online. Additionally, she is an attorney with 20 years' experience in combining nursing and the law. She is frequently a guest speaker on legal issues in nursing education and has authored multiple chapters on nursing law for various nursing education books.

Larry E. Simmons, PhD, RN, CNE, NEA-BC is the Director of the Certification Program at the National League for Nursing. He received an associate's degree in nursing from Metropolitan Community College, a bachelor's degree from the University of Missouri–Kansas City, as well as a master's in nursing and his doctorate degrees. Dr. Simmons is widely known for his expertise in nursing education and in standardized testing, along with the psychometrics of testing results. He has been a nurse educator for more than 20 years as well as serving as a consultant to many 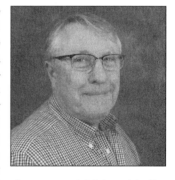 programs of nursing across the United States. He also has a special interest in the global community of nursing education, traveling internationally to promote certification for nurse educators. He has been active in many professional nursing organizations, including the American Assembly of Men in Nursing and Sigma Theta Tau, International. Representing the certification program at the NLN, he is also involved in the American Board of Nursing Specialties group.

Contents

1

The Development of the Academic Nurse Educator Scope of Practice and the Academic Clinical Nurse Educator Scope of Practice

INTRODUCTION

The purpose of this book is to describe academic nursing education and academic clinical nursing education as specialty areas and advanced nursing practice roles within professional nursing. The historical perspective, values and beliefs, theoretical framework, research in the academic nurse educator role(s), and future for the academic nurse educator roles are presented. The discussion of each role includes definitions, scope of practice, standards of practice, and specific competencies.

The Scope of Practice for Academic Nurse Educators was first developed by the Certification Governance Committee of the National League for Nursing (NLN) and published by the NLN in 2005. At that time, the leadership of the NLN and the members of the committee believed that recognition of academic nursing education as a specialty and an advanced nursing practice role was essential. They also determined that a description of the scope and competencies of nurse educator practice and a certification exam linked to those competencies were required.

During 2010 and 2011, the NLN's Certification Commission collaborated to perform an updated nurse educator practice analysis. This systematic practice analysis assessment was intended to identify any changes in the job-related responsibilities of individuals who fulfill the full scope of the nurse faculty role. The results of the 2010 to 2011 practice analysis resulted in slight revisions to the nurse educator certification test blueprint. The nurse educator practice analysis was performed again in 2016 and 2017, also resulting in minor revisions to the nurse educator certification test blueprint.

The academic nurse educator competencies first identified pertained to the faculty member who was practicing in the full scope of the nurse educator role. However, not all academic nurse educators practice in the full scope of the nurse educator role. Some nurse educators focus their practice in the clinical setting. As of 2015, the role of the academic clinical nurse educator had not been described, nor had its competencies been identified. The NLN created a task group to identify the core competencies of this specific role. A practice analysis was conducted in 2016 and 2017 on the role of the academic clinical nurse educator; the results were instrumental in creating the test plan for a new certification as an NLN Academic Clinical Nurse Educator.

HISTORICAL PERSPECTIVE

The development of educational programs for the preparation of nurses parallels the evolution of nursing as a distinct profession requiring a specialized body of knowledge and skills. One of the earliest known training programs was the Deaconess Institute established in Kaiserswerth, Germany, in 1836. Deaconesses were women who promised to work for Christ by teaching or nursing. The institute became well known, and graduates of the program spread the Kaiserswerth model of care of the ill throughout the world (Donahue, 1996).

Florence Nightingale trained at the Kaiserswerth Institute in 1851. On her return to England from the Crimea in 1856, Nightingale set about achieving her two key goals: "reform of army sanitary practices and the establishment of a school for nurses" (Kalisch & Kalisch, 1995, p. 36). Today, Nightingale is credited with defining a theoretical foundation for the practice of nursing and founding the first independent organized training program for nurses (Donahue, 1996).

In the United States, the mid-nineteenth century saw calls for formal training of nurses by organizations such as the American Medical Association. The first training school for nurses in America was established in 1872 at New England Hospital.

By 1902, there were 492 schools of nursing in the United States. Training programs expected strict discipline, long hours, and a strong focus on learning through practice. Programs began to expand from two to three years and schools known for their high quality of training attracted students of increasing caliber. In 1905, Bellevue Hospital had 2,000 applicants (Kalisch & Kalisch, 1995).

During the early twentieth century, most nurses were prepared in hospital-based programs. However, starting with the University of Minnesota in 1909, collegiate settings became the locus for programs of registered nursing education at the undergraduate and graduate levels. The approach to providing registered nursing education in community colleges was developed by Dr. Mildred Montag in 1949.

During this period and beyond, several important studies guided the evolution of nursing education. In 1923, the first evaluation of nursing education, by Goldmark, was published. Examples of other key documents include *Nurses, Patients, and Pocketbooks* (1923), *Nursing Schools Today and Tomorrow* (1934), *Nursing for the Future* (1948), *Nurses for a Growing Nation* (1957), *Toward Quality in Nursing* (1961), *ANA Position Paper on Education for Nursing* (1965), and *Extending the Scope of Nursing Practice* (1971) (Kalisch & Kalisch, 1995). These documents provided important guidance to the development of nursing education in the United States and Canada.

As nursing progressed to become a profession, the science of nursing was further delineated. In addition, the body of knowledge and skills unique to generalist and advanced practice nursing was developed and refined. Preparation of professional nurses transitioned from "training" to "education."

The first organization for nursing in the United States was officially developed in 1893. The American Society of Superintendents of Training Schools of Nurses (ASSTSN) was formed for "the establishment and maintenance of a universal standard of training" for nursing (Fondiller, 1999). The ASSTSN evolved into the National League for Nursing Education (NLNE) in 1912 and then the National League for Nursing in 1952.

The first formal training programs for practical nurses were started by the Brooklyn YMCA in 1893. However, the first school was not organized until 1897.

The shortage of nurses that followed World War II prompted the expansion of practical nurse (PN) programs, with most housed in public schools. The practical nurse programs of today are commonly one year in length, and most PN education takes place in vocational/technical schools and community colleges (Kelly & Joel, 1996).

Although nursing education has existed for more than 160 years, academic nursing education as a specialty area of practice with a defined theoretical basis, body of knowledge, and certification has been slow to develop. Preparation of nurses as educators has occurred in graduate programs of nursing or education or through continuing education, mentoring, or experience. In order to further advance nursing education, new models of research-based nursing education must emerge. The precedent of relying on tradition and past practices must be replaced with proposed changes emanating from "evidence that substantiates the science of nursing education and provides the foundation for best educational practices" (NLN, 2005b, p. 1).

VALUES AND BELIEFS

Academic nurse educators believe that education is a self-actualizing, creative, lifetime endeavor involving values clarification, progressive systematic inquiry, critical analysis, and judgment.

As a distinct specialty of advanced nursing practice, academic nursing education has a set of defined values and beliefs. They are evident in the *NLN Hallmarks of Excellence in Nursing Education*© (outlined in the following section) and are incorporated into the standards of practice. The Hallmarks were originally published in 2004 and revised in 2019. The Hallmarks are relevant for all types of nursing programs and all types of institutions.

NLN HALLMARKS OF EXCELLENCE IN NURSING EDUCATION©

Hallmark # 1-1–Engaged Students

Students are excited about learning and exhibit a spirit of inquiry as well as a commitment to lifelong learning.

Hallmark # 1-2–Engaged Students

Students are committed to innovation, continuous quality/performance improvement, and excellence.

Hallmark # 1-3–Engaged Students

Students are committed to the professional nursing role, including advancement in leadership, scholarship, and mentoring.

Hallmark # 2-1–Diverse, Well-Prepared Faculty

The faculty complement is comprised of diverse individuals who are leaders, and/or have expertise in clinical practice, education, interprofessional collaboration, and research/scholarship consistent with the parent institution's mission and vision.

Hallmark # 2-2–Diverse, Well-Prepared Faculty

The unique contributions of each faculty member in teaching, service, research/scholarship, and practice that facilitate achievement of the program's mission and goals are valued, rewarded, and recognized.

Hallmark # 2-3–Diverse, Well-Prepared Faculty

Faculty members are accountable for promoting excellence, creating civil and inclusive environments, and providing leadership in their area(s) of expertise.

Hallmark # 2-4–Diverse, Well-Prepared Faculty

Faculty members model a commitment to lifelong learning, involvement in professional and community organizations, and scholarly activities.

Hallmark # 2-5–Diverse, Well-Prepared Faculty

All faculty members have structured preparation for the faculty role, including competence in teaching, scholarship, and service.

Hallmark # 3-1–A Culture of Continuous Quality Improvement

The program engages in a variety of activities that promote quality and excellence, including accreditation by national nursing accreditation bodies.

Hallmark # 3-2–A Culture of Continuous Quality Improvement

Program design, implementation, and evaluation are continuously reviewed and revised to achieve and maintain excellence.

Hallmark # 4-1–Innovative, Evidence-Based Curriculum

The curriculum is designed to help students achieve stated program outcomes, reflects current societal and health care trends and issues, and is responsive to change and evolving societal needs. The curriculum also embeds evidence-based information, reflects research findings and innovative practices, attends to the evolving role of the nurse in a variety of settings, is flexible, is innovative, and incorporates local, national, and global perspectives.

Hallmark # 4-2–Innovative, Evidence-Based Curriculum

The curriculum provides learning activities that enhance students' abilities to think critically, reflect thoughtfully, and provide culturally sensitive, evidence-based nursing care to diverse populations.

Hallmark # 4-3–Innovative, Evidence-Based Curriculum

The curriculum emphasizes students' values development, identity formation, caring for self, commitment to lifelong learning, critical thinking, ethical and evidence-based practice, and creativity.

Hallmark # 4-4–Innovative, Evidence-Based Curriculum

The curriculum provides learning experiences that prepare graduates to assume roles that are essential to quality nursing practice, including but not limited to roles of care provider, advocate for those in need, teacher, communicator, change agent, care coordinator, member of intra- and inter-professional teams, user of information technology, collaborator, decision-maker, leader, and evolving scholar.

Hallmark # 4-5–Innovative, Evidence-Based Curriculum

The curriculum provides learning experiences that support evidence-based practice, interprofessional approaches to care, student achievement of clinical competence, and, as appropriate, competence in a specialty role.

Hallmark # 5-1–Innovative, Evidence-Based Approaches to Facilitate and Evaluate Learning

Strategies used to facilitate and evaluate learning by a diverse student population are innovative and varied.

Hallmark # 5-2–Innovative, Evidence-Based Approaches to Facilitate and Evaluate Learning

Faculty members engage in collegial dialogue and interact with students and colleagues in nursing and other professions to promote and develop strategies to facilitate and evaluate learning.

Hallmark # 5-3–Innovative, Evidence-Based Approaches to Facilitate and Evaluate Learning

Strategies to facilitate and evaluate learning used by faculty members are evidence-based.

Hallmark # 6-1–Resources to Support Program Goal Attainment

Partnerships in which the program is engaged promote excellence in nursing education, enhance the profession, benefit the community, enhance learning opportunities, and facilitate/support research/scholarship initiatives.

Hallmark # 6-2–Resources to Support Program Goal Attainment

Technology is used effectively to facilitate, support, and evaluate student learning; faculty development; research/scholarship; and support services.

Hallmark # 6-3–Resources to Support Program Goal Attainment

Student support services are culturally sensitive and empower students during the recruitment, retention, progression, graduation, and career planning processes.

Hallmark # 6-4–Resources to Support Program Goal Attainment

Financial resources are available to support initiatives that enhance faculty competence, student success, innovation, and scholarly endeavors.

Hallmark # 7-1–Commitment to Pedagogical Scholarship

Faculty members and students contribute to the development of the science of nursing education through the critique, use, dissemination, and/or conduct of various forms of scholarly endeavors.

Hallmark # 7-2–Commitment to Pedagogical Scholarship

Faculty members and students explore the influence of student learning experiences on the health of the individuals and populations they serve in various health care settings.

Hallmark # 8-1–Effective Institutional and Professional Leadership

Faculty members, administrators, and students provide the leadership needed to ensure that the culture of the school promotes excellence and a healthy work environment characterized by collegial dialogue, innovation, change, creativity, values development, and ethical behavior.

Hallmark # 8-2–Effective Institutional and Professional Leadership

Faculty members, administrators, students, and alumni are respected as leaders in the parent institution, as well as in local, state, regional, national, and/or international communities.

Hallmark # 8-3–Effective Institutional and Professional Leadership

Faculty members, administrators, students, and alumni are prepared for and assume leadership roles that advance quality nursing care; promote positive change, innovation, and excellence; and enhance the impact of the nursing profession.

THEORETICAL FOUNDATIONS

Nursing: Scope and Standards of Practice, Third Edition (American Nurses Association [ANA], 2015) builds on previous work and provides the following contemporary definition of nursing: "Nursing is the protection, promotion, and optimization of health and abilities, prevention of illness and injury, facilitation of healing, alleviation of suffering through the diagnosis and treatment of human response, and advocacy in the care of individuals, families, groups, communities, and populations" (ANA, 2015, p. 7).

As a specialty area of advanced nursing practice, academic nursing education has a theoretical foundation that includes models and theories from nursing science, "educational psychology, instructional technology, instructional design, tests and measurement, and evaluation theory" (Caputi & Engelmann, 2004, p. 3).

Several models and theories have been used to develop the scope and standards of practice in the academic nurse educator role that are relevant to faculty teaching in all types of nursing programs: practical nurse, associate degree, diploma, baccalaureate, master's, and doctoral. Examples of models and theories from education with relevance for nursing education include Boyer's scholarship of engagement (Boyer, 1990), Kolb's learning cycle (Kolb, 1984), Bloom's taxonomy of learning objectives (Krathwol, Bloom, & Masia, 1964), learning theories such as Knowles's adult learning theory (Knowles, Holton, & Swanson, 1998), community-academic partnerships (Tagliareni & Marckx, 1997), and service-learning (Community Campus Partnerships for Health, n.d.).

Boyer (1990) described a perspective of the scholarly role of faculty that went beyond the traditional interpretation of research as the "only way to increase the knowledge of the discipline and as the only means for incentive and compensation of the academic professional" (Kirkpatrick & Valley, 2004). He outlined four types of scholarship in which faculty engage: discovery (disciplined investigative efforts leading to new knowledge), integration (synthesis, making connections across disciplines), application (using knowledge in implementing a practice role or in service to the larger community), and teaching (transmitting, transforming, and extending knowledge). The extent to which a particular academic nurse educator engages in each type of scholarship will vary in accord with factors such as her/his professional goals and the type of program in which she/he teaches.

The Academic Nurse Educator Practicing in the Full Scope of the Role

2

DEFINITION

Academic nursing education is the process of facilitating learning through curriculum design, teaching, evaluation, advisement, and other activities undertaken by faculty in schools of nursing. Academic nursing education is a specialty area and an advanced practice role within professional nursing.

Academic nurse educators engage in a number of roles and functions, each of which reflects the core competencies of nursing faculty. The extent to which a specific nurse educator implements these competencies varies according to many factors, including the mission of the nurse educator's institution, the nurse educator's academic rank, the nurse educator's academic preparation, and the type of program in which the nurse educator teaches. The academic nurse educator engaged in all of the core competencies is considered to be practicing in the full scope of the role.

SCOPE OF PRACTICE

"The scope of practice statement describes the 'who, what, where, when, why, and how' of nursing practice" (ANA, 2017, p. 14). The term "academic nurse educator" refers to an individual who fulfills a faculty role in an academic setting. In nursing, this role is implemented in practical nurse (PN), registered nurse (RN), and graduate programs.

Whereas individuals with appointments to a nursing faculty may hold advanced preparation in disciplines supportive to nursing (e.g., nutrition, pharmacology), the scope of practice described here relates to individuals with advanced preparation in nursing who teach nursing courses. "Competence as an educator can be established, recognized, and expanded through master's and/or doctoral education, post-master's certificate programs, continuing professional development, mentoring activities, and professional certification as a faculty member" (NLN, 2002, p. 4).

Nursing education takes place in diverse settings that include, but are not limited to, technical schools, hospitals, two- and four-year colleges, and universities. The implementation of the academic faculty role may occur in traditional classroom-based environments or in nontraditional environments.

Academic nurse educators engage in a number of roles and functions, each of which reflects the core competencies of nursing faculty. The NLN (2005a) identified nurse educator competencies as the following: (1) facilitate learning, (2) facilitate learner development and socialization, (3) use assessment and evaluation strategies, (4) participate in curriculum design and evaluation of program outcomes, (5) function as a change agent and leader, (6) pursue continuous quality improvement in the nurse educator role, (7) engage in scholarship, and (8) function within the educational environment. The extent to which a specific nurse educator implements these competencies varies according to many factors, including the mission of the educator's institution, rank, academic preparation, and type of program in which the educator is teaching.

The development of a master nurse educator evolves over time. To that end, it is recognized that many nurse educators function at a competent level early in their careers, but mastery occurs with guidance, ongoing professional development, and practice.

STANDARDS OF PRACTICE

Standards of practice are considered authoritative duties that nurses are expected to perform competently (ANA, 2017). The ANA further identified two categorizes of standards: "a) Standards of Practice that describe a competent level of nursing practice as demonstrated by the nursing process, and b) Standards of Professional Performance that describe a competent level of behavior in the professional role" (p. 4).

An academic nurse educator is a professional role within nursing. The core competencies set out in the next section identify the diverse duties that have become the standards of professional role performance for academic nurse educators practicing in the full scope of the role.

CORE COMPETENCIES OF ACADEMIC NURSE EDUCATORS© WITH TASK STATEMENTS

Competency I: Facilitate Learning

Nurse educators are responsible for creating an environment in classroom, laboratory, and clinical settings that facilitates student learning and the achievement of desired cognitive, affective, and psychomotor outcomes. To facilitate learning effectively, the nurse educator:

› Implements a variety of teaching strategies appropriate to learner needs, desired learner outcomes, content, and context

› Grounds teaching strategies in educational theory and evidence-based teaching practices

> Recognizes multicultural, gender, and experiential influences on teaching and learning
> Engages in self-reflection and continued learning to improve teaching practices that facilitate learning
> Uses information technologies skillfully to support the teaching-learning process
> Practices skilled oral, written, and electronic communication that reflects an awareness of self and others, along with an ability to convey ideas in a variety of contexts
> Models critical and reflective thinking
> Creates opportunities for learners to develop their critical thinking and critical reasoning skills
> Shows enthusiasm for teaching, learning, and nursing that inspires and motivates students
> Demonstrates interest in and respect for learners
> Uses personal attributes (e.g., caring, confidence, patience, integrity, and flexibility) that facilitate learning
> Develops collegial working relationships with students, faculty colleagues, and clinical agency personnel to promote positive learning environments
> Maintains the professional practice knowledge base needed to help learners prepare for contemporary nursing practice
> Serves as a role model of professional nursing

Competency II: Facilitate Learner Development and Socialization

Nurse educators recognize the responsibility for helping students develop as nurses and integrate the values and behaviors expected of those who fulfill that role. To facilitate learner development and formation effectively, the nurse educator:

> Identifies individual learning styles and unique learning needs of international, adult, multicultural, educationally disadvantaged, physically challenged, at-risk, and second-degree learners
> Provides resources to diverse learners that help meet their individual learning needs
> Engages in effective advisement and counseling strategies that help learners meet their professional goals
> Creates learning environments that are focused on socialization to the role of the nurse and facilitate learners' self-reflection and personal goal setting
> Fosters the cognitive, psychomotor, and affective development of learners
> Recognizes the influence of teaching styles and interpersonal interactions on learner outcomes

▸ Assists learners to develop the ability to engage in thoughtful and constructive self- and peer evaluation

▸ Models professional behaviors for learners including, but not limited to, involvement in professional organizations, engagement in lifelong learning activities, dissemination of information through publications and presentations, and advocacy

Competency III: Use Assessment and Evaluation Strategies

Nurse educators use a variety of strategies to assess and evaluate student learning in classroom, laboratory and clinical settings, as well as in all domains of learning. To use assessment and evaluation strategies effectively, the nurse educator:

▸ Uses extant literature to develop evidence-based assessment and evaluation practices

▸ Uses a variety of strategies to assess and evaluate learning in the cognitive, psychomotor, and affective domains

▸ Implements evidence-based assessment and evaluation strategies that are appropriate to the learner and to learning goals

▸ Uses assessment and evaluation data to enhance the teaching-learning process

▸ Provides timely, constructive, and thoughtful feedback to learners

▸ Demonstrates skill in the design and use of tools for assessing clinical practice

Competency IV: Participate in Curriculum Design and Evaluation of Program Outcomes

Nurse educators are responsible for formulating program outcomes and designing curricula that reflect contemporary health care trends and prepare graduates to function effectively in the health care environment. To participate effectively in curriculum design and systematic evaluation of program outcomes, the nurse educator:

▸ Ensures that the curriculum reflects institutional philosophy and mission, current nursing and health care trends, and community and societal needs so as to prepare graduates for practice in a complex, dynamic, multicultural health care environment

▸ Demonstrates knowledge of curriculum development, including identifying program outcomes, developing competency statements, writing learning objectives, and selecting appropriate learning activities and evaluation strategies

▸ Bases curriculum design and implementation decisions on sound educational principles, theory, and research

▸ Revises the curriculum based on assessment of program outcomes, learner needs, and societal and health care trends

> Implements curricular revisions using appropriate change theories and strategies

> Creates and maintains community and clinical partnerships that support educational goals

> Collaborates with external constituencies throughout the process of curriculum revision

> Designs and implements program assessment models that promote continuous quality improvement of all aspects of the program

Competency V: Function as a Change Agent and Leader

Nurse educators function as change agents and leaders to create a preferred future for nursing education and nursing practice. To function effectively as a change agent and leader, the nurse educator:

> Models cultural sensitivity when advocating for change

> Integrates a long-term, innovative, and creative perspective into the nurse educator role

> Participates in interdisciplinary efforts to address health care and educational needs locally, regionally, nationally, or internationally

> Evaluates organizational effectiveness in nursing education

> Implements strategies for organizational change

> Provides leadership in the parent institution as well as in the nursing program to enhance the visibility of nursing and its contributions to the academic community

> Promotes innovative practices in educational environments

> Develops leadership skills to shape and implement change

Competency VI: Pursue Continuous Quality Improvement in the Nurse Educator Role

Nurse educators recognize that their role is multidimensional and that an ongoing commitment to develop and maintain competence in the role is essential. To pursue continuous quality improvement in the nurse educator role, the individual:

> Demonstrates a commitment to lifelong learning

> Recognizes that career enhancement needs and activities change as experience is gained in the role

> Participates in professional development opportunities that increase one's effectiveness in the role

> Balances the teaching, scholarship, and service demands inherent in the role of educator and member of an academic institution

> Uses feedback gained from self, peer, student, and administrative evaluation to improve role effectiveness

> Engages in activities that promote one's socialization to the role

> Uses knowledge of legal and ethical issues relevant to higher education and nursing education as a basis for influencing, designing, and implementing policies and procedures related to students, faculty, and the educational environment

> Mentors and supports faculty colleagues

Competency VII: Engage in Scholarship

Nurse educators acknowledge that scholarship is an integral component of the faculty role, and that teaching itself is a scholarly activity. To engage effectively in scholarship, the nurse educator:

> Draws on extant literature to design evidence-based teaching and evaluation practices

> Exhibits a spirit of inquiry about teaching and learning, student development, evaluation methods, and other aspects of the role

> Designs and implements scholarly activities in an established area of expertise

> Disseminates nursing and teaching knowledge to a variety of audiences through various means

> Demonstrates skill in proposal writing for initiatives that include, but are not limited to, research, resource acquisition, program development, and policy development

> Demonstrates qualities of a scholar: integrity, courage, perseverance, vitality, and creativity

Competency VIII: Function Within the Educational Environment

Nurse educators are knowledgeable about the educational environment within which they practice and recognize how political, institutional, social, and economic forces impact their role. To function as a good "citizen of the academy," the nurse educator:

> Uses knowledge of history and current trends and issues in higher education as a basis for making recommendations and decisions on educational issues

> Identifies how social, economic, political, and institutional forces influence higher education in general and nursing education in particular

> Develops networks, collaborations, and partnerships to enhance nursing's influence within the academic community

> Determines own professional goals within the context of academic nursing and the mission of the parent institution and nursing program

> Integrates the values of respect, collegiality, professionalism, and caring to build an organizational climate that fosters the development of students and teachers
> Incorporates the goals of the nursing program and the mission of the parent institution when proposing change or managing issues
> Assumes a leadership role in various levels of institutional governance
> Advocates for nursing and nursing education in the political arena

3

The Academic Clinical Nurse Educator Practicing Within the Clinical Educator Role

DEFINITION

According to the *NLN Certified Academic Clinical Nurse Educator (CNE®cl) 2019 Candidate Handbook,* "the academic clinical nurse educator facilitates the learning of nursing students throughout clinical components of an academic nursing program. This educator is guided in this role by faculty of the nursing program and is accountable to that nursing program for providing fair evaluations of learners' performance in meeting expected learning outcomes. The academic clinical nurse educator may have a variety of titles depending upon the classification used by the specific nursing education program (e.g., clinical faculty, part-time faculty, adjunct faculty, clinical instructor, preceptor)" (NLN, 2019, p. 2).

SCOPE OF PRACTICE

The academic clinical nurse educator has experience within professional nursing practice and academic nursing education practice. Within professional nursing practice, the academic clinical nurse educator has gained competence in nursing practice and can share this competence with students in the clinical components of academic nursing education.

The academic clinical nurse educator also "has experience as an educator in an academic setting and responsibility for facilitating student learning (in the classroom, laboratory, and/or clinical setting), and the educator experience may be with learners enrolled in pre- or post-licensure nursing programs" (NLN, 2019, p. 2).

The academic clinical nurse educator's role varies from other clinical educator roles, such as the traditional hospital-based clinical nurse educator who provides employee orientation and staff development. The academic clinical nurse educator "reports to a school/department of nursing about learner performance in clinical settings, submits evaluations about the performance of learners receiving academic credit for the clinical learning experience, and supervises the learner in the setting" (NLN, 2019, p. 2). This role is accountable for selecting appropriate clinical learning experiences and providing support for the learner to meet the expected clinical outcomes.

STANDARDS OF PRACTICE

The academic clinical nurse educator is a professional role within nursing. The core competencies set out in the next section reflect the standards of professional role performance for the academic clinical nurse educator.

CORE COMPETENCIES OF ACADEMIC CLINICAL NURSE EDUCATORS© WITH TASK STATEMENTS

Competency I: Function Within the Education and Health Care Environments

A. Function in the Clinical Educator Role.

> Bridge the gap between theory and practice by helping learners apply classroom learning to the clinical setting.

> Foster professional growth of learners.

> Use technologies to enhance clinical teaching and learning.

> Value the contributions of others in the achievement of learner outcomes.

> Act as a role model of professional nursing within the clinical learning environment.

> Demonstrate inclusive excellence.

B. Operationalize the Curriculum.

> Assess congruence of the clinical agency to the curriculum, core goals, and learner needs.

> Plan meaningful and relevant clinical learning assignments and activities.

> Identify learners' goals and outcomes.

> Prepare learners for clinical experiences.

> Structure learner experiences within the learning environment to promote optimal learning.

> Implement clinical learning activities to help learners develop interprofessional collaboration and teamwork skills.

> Provide opportunities for learners to develop problem-solving and clinical reasoning skills related to learning outcomes.

> Implement assigned models for clinical teaching.

> Engage in theory-based instruction.

> Provide input to the nursing program for course development and review.

C. Abide by Legal Requirements, Ethical Guidelines, Agency Policies, and Guiding Framework.

> Apply ethical and legal principles to create a safe clinical learning environment.

> Assess learner abilities and needs prior to clinical learning experiences.

> Facilitate learning activities that support the mission, goals, and values of the academic institution and the clinical agency.

> Inform others of program and clinical agency policies, procedures, and practices.

> Adhere to program and clinical agency policies, procedures, and practices when implementing clinical experiences.

> Promote learner compliance with regulations and standards of practice.

> Demonstrate ethical behaviors.

Competency II: Facilitate Learning in the Health Care Environment

> Implement a variety of clinical teaching strategies congruent with learner needs, desired learner outcomes, content, and context.

> Ground teaching strategies in educational theory and evidence-based teaching practices.

> Use technology skillfully to support the teaching-learning process.

> Create opportunities for learners to develop critical thinking and clinical reasoning skills.

> Promote a culture of safety and quality in the health care environment.

> Create a positive and caring learning environment.

> Develop collegial working relationships with learners, faculty colleagues, and clinical agency personnel.

> Demonstrate enthusiasm for teaching, learning, and nursing to help inspire and motivate learners.

Competency III: Demonstrate Effective Interpersonal Communication and Collaborative Interprofessional Relationships

> Value collaboration and coordination of care.

> Foster a shared learning community and cooperate with other members of the health care team.

> Support an environment of frequent, respectful, civil, and open communication with all members of the health care team.

> Act as a role model, showing respect for all members of the health care team, professional colleagues, clients, family members, as well as learners.

> Use clear and effective communication in all interactions.

> Listen to learner concerns, needs, or questions in a nonthreatening way.

> Display a calm, empathetic, and supportive demeanor in all communications.

> Manage emotions effectively when communicating in challenging situations.

> Effectively manage conflict.

> Maintain an approachable, nonjudgmental, and readily accessible demeanor.

> Recognize limitations in self and learners to provide opportunities for development.

> Demonstrate effective communication in clinical learning environments with diverse colleagues, clients, cultures, health care professionals, and learners.

> Communicate performance expectations to learners and agency staff.

Competency IV: Applies Clinical Expertise in the Health Care Environment

> Maintain current professional competence relevant to the specialty area, practice setting, and clinical learning environment.

> Translate theory into clinical practice by applying experiential knowledge, clinical reasoning, and using a client-centered approach to clinical instruction.

> Use best evidence to address client-related problems.

> Demonstrate effective leadership within the clinical learning environment.

> Demonstrate sound clinical reasoning.

> Expand knowledge and skills by integrating best practices.

> Balance client care needs and student learning needs within a culture of safety.

> Demonstrate competence with a range of technologies available in the clinical learning environment.

Competency V: Facilitate Learner Development and Socialization

> Mentor learners in the development of professional nursing behaviors, standards, and codes of ethics.

> Promote a learning climate of respect for all.

> Promote professional integrity and accountability.

> Maintain professional boundaries.

> Encourage ongoing learner professional development via formal and informal venues.
> Assist learners in effective use of self-assessment and professional goal setting for ongoing self-improvement.
> Create learning environments that are focused on socialization to the role of the nurse.
> Assist learners to develop the ability to engage in constructive peer feedback.
> Inspire creativity and confidence.
> Encourage various techniques for learners to develop the ability to engage in constructive peer feedback.
> Inspire creativity and confidence.
> Encourage various techniques for learners to manage stress.
> Act as a role model for self-reflection, self-care, and coping skills.
> Empower learners to be successful in meeting professional and educational goals.
> Engage learners in applying best practices and quality improvement processes.

Competency VI: Implement Effective Clinical and Assessment Evaluation Strategies

> Use a variety of strategies to determine achievement of learning outcomes.
> Implement both formative and summative evaluation that is appropriate to the learner and learner outcomes.
> Engage in timely communication with course faculty regarding learner clinical performance.
> Maintain integrity in the assessment and evaluation of learners.
> Provide timely, objective, constructive, and fair feedback to learners.
> Use learner data to enhance the teaching-learning process in the clinical learning environment.
> Demonstrate skill in the use of best practices in the assessment and evaluation of clinical performance.
> Assess and evaluate learner achievement of clinical performance expectations.
> Use performance standards to determine learner strengths and weaknesses in the clinical learning environment.
> Document learner clinical performance, feedback, and progression.
> Evaluate the quality of the clinical learning experiences and environment.

4

Literature Focused on the Role of the Academic Nurse Educator and Academic Clinical Nurse Educator

Since the NLN identified the core competencies of the academic nurse educator in 2005, the competencies have been integrated within nursing education in various ways. The competencies have been the basis for promoting education within the faculty role through their integration into graduate nursing education curricula and nursing faculty continuing education offerings (Christensen & Halstead, 2019). The NLN academic nurse educator competencies have also been integrated into the position descriptions of nurse educators and their performance evaluations (Christensen & Halstead, 2019). Use of the core competencies as the framework for nurse educator orientation programs was suggested by Danna, Schaubhut, and Jones (2010).

Despite the use of the NLN academic nurse educator competencies, little research has been conducted related to this role or the competencies (Christensen, 2015). Such research can be identified as qualitative studies, studies focusing on CNE exam outcomes, descriptive studies of perceived competence of nurse educators, and quasi-experimental studies (Frenn & Dreifuerst, 2019).

The NLN core competencies of the academic clinical nurse educator have only recently been identified. As a result, very little can be found in the literature focused on the academic clinical nurse educator competencies, and no research related to these competencies can be identified.

The NLN's research agenda promotes the role of nurse scientists and calls for nurse scholars to "build the science of nursing education through the discovery and translation of innovative evidence-based strategies." Future research related to the academic nurse educator competencies and academic clinical nurse educator competencies could focus on answering questions such as: does faculty competency attainment impact faculty performance and student outcomes, do self-ratings of certified nurse educators correlate significantly with interrater evaluated ratings as to attainment of core competencies, or what are the priority competencies for nurse educators teaching in a variety of different program types (Frenn & Dreifuerst, 2019). Academic clinical nurse educator competency research could initially focus on descriptive studies of those who attain certification and qualitative studies.

A limited number of publications, both research and nonresearch, have been included in the NLN's research journal *Nursing Education Perspectives* (NEP). A summary of the NEP publications is included in Appendix A. The NEP publications focused on the academic nurse educator role and certification include article abstracts, President's Message, and NEP Quick Reads and Headlines from the NLN.

The Future for Academic Nurse Educator Roles: Final Thoughts

5

Nursing education is a dynamic field that is experiencing the challenges of a nursing faculty shortage, increasingly sophisticated technologies, and the stimulation of a diverse student population. Clinical competence and educational expertise are required to continue the advancement of our specialty. The influence of evidence-based practice and new research in nursing education, successful collaboration with other disciplines, and mentorship of new faculty colleagues make it imperative that the scope of practice for academic nurse educator roles remains dynamic and continues to evolve. This third edition addressing the scope of practice for academic nurse educator roles is evidence of the dynamic evolution of the academic faculty roles.

References

American Nurses Association. (2015). *Nursing scope and standards of practice* (3rd ed.). Retrieved from https://www.iupuc.edu/health-sciences/files/Nursing-Scope Standards-3E.pdf

American Nurses Association. (2017). American Nurses Association recognition of a nursing specialty, approval of a specialty nursing scope of practice statement, acknowledgment of specialty nursing standards of practice, and affirmation of focused practice competencies. Retrieved from https://www.nursingworld.org/~4989de/globalassets/practiceandpolicy/scope-of-practice/3sc-booklet-final-2017-08-17.pdf

Boyer, E. (1990). *Scholarship reconsidered: Priorities of the professoriate*. Princeton, NJ: Carnegie Foundation for the Advancement of Teaching.

Caputi, L., & Engelmann, L. (2004). *Teaching nursing: The art and science*. Glen Ellyn, IL: College of DuPage Press.

Christensen, L. S. (2015). *Factors related to success on the Certified Nurse Educator (CNE) examination (Doctoral dissertation)*. Retrieved from ProQuest Dissertations and Theses database. (Accession No. 3708579).

Christensen, L. S., & Halstead, J. A. (2019). The influence of the core competencies for nurse educators: 2005–2015. In J. A. Halstead (Ed.), *NLN core competencies for nurse educators: A decade of influence*. Washington, DC: National League for Nursing.

Community Campus Partnerships for Health. (n.d.). Retrieved from https://www.ccphealth.org

Danna, D. M., Schaubhut, R. M., & Jones, J. R. (2010). From practice to education: Perspectives from three nurse leaders. *Journal of Continuing Nursing Education*, *41*(2), 83–87.

Donahue, M. P. (1996). *Nursing, the finest art: An illustrated history* (2nd ed.). St. Louis, MO: Mosby.

Frenn, M., & Dreifuerst, K. (2019). Summary of research using the NLN core competencies of nurse educators as a framework. In J. A. Halstead (Ed.), *NLN core competencies for nurse educators: A decade of influence*. Washington, DC: National League for Nursing.

Fondiller, S. H. (1999). One hundred years ago: Nursing education at the dawn of the 20th century [From the archives]. *Nursing and Health Care Perspectives*, *20*(6), 286–288.

Kalisch, P., & Kalisch, B. (1995). *The advance of American nursing* (3rd ed.). Philadelphia, PA: J. B. Lippincott.

Kelly, L. Y., & Joel, L. A. (1996). *The nursing experience: Trends, challenges, and transitions* (3rd ed.). New York, NY: McGraw-Hill.

Kirkpatrick, J., & Valley, J. (2004). Finding success in the faculty role. In L. Caputi & L. Englemann (Eds.), *Teaching nursing: The art and science* (pp. 972–989). Glenn Ellyn, IL: College of DuPage Press.

Knowles, M., Holton, E., & Swanson, R. (1998). *The adult learner: The definitive classic in adult education and human resource development* (5th ed.). Houston, TX: Gulf.

Kolb, D. A. (1984). *Experiential learning: Experience as a source of learning and development*. Englewood Cliffs, NJ: Prentice-Hall.

Krathwol, D. R., Bloom, B. S., & Masia, B. (1964). *Taxonomy of educational objectives, Handbook II*. New York, NY: David McKay.

National League for Nursing (2002). The preparation of nurse educators [Archived Position Statement]. Retrieved from http://www.nln.org/docs/default-source/about/archived-position-statements/the-preparation-of-nurse-educators-pdf.pdf?sfvrsn=6

National League for Nursing. (2005a). *The scope of practice for academic nurse educators*. New York, NY: Author.

National League for Nursing. (2005b). Transforming nursing education [Archived Position Statement]. Retrieved from http://www.nln.org/docs/default-source/about/archived-position-statements/transforming052009.pdf?sfvrsn=6

National League for Nursing. (2019). *NLN certified academic clinical nurse educator (CNE®cl) 2018 candidate handbook*. Retrieved from http://www.nln.org/Certification-for-Nurse-Educators/cnecl/cne-cl-handbook

National League for Nursing (2019a). Mission and strategic plan 2019–2021. Retrieved from http://www.nln.org/about/mission-goals

National League for Nursing (2019b). *Hallmarks of excellence: Hallmarks, indicators, glossary & references*. Retrieved from http://www.nln.org/professional-development-programs/teaching-resources/hallmarks-of-excellence

Tagliareni, M. E., & Marckx, B. (1997). *Teaching in the community: Preparing nurses for the 21st century*. New York, NY: National League for Nursing.

Nursing Education Perspectives Publications Focused on the Certified Nurse Educator Role

NEP ABSTRACTS

Defining the Professional Responsibilities of Academic Nurse Educators: The Results of a National Practice Analysis

Tracy A. Ortelli, MS, RN

Abstract

In February 2005, the National League for Nursing's Academic Nurse Educator Certification Program and its testing service partner, Applied Measurement Professionals, Inc. (AMP), conducted a study designed to determine the professional practice responsibilities of academic nurse educators. The results of this national practice analysis, reported here, provided the initial information required to ensure the development of a practice-related, content-valid certification examination for academic nurse educators. [**Nursing Education Perspectives**, 27(5), 242–246, September/October 2006]

From Committee to Commission: The History of the NLN's Academic Certified Nurse Educator Program

Jan M. Nick, PhD, RNC-OB, CNE, ANEF; Nancy C. Sharts-Hopko, PhD, RN, CNE, FAAN; and Debra Woodard Leners, PhD, RN, PNP, CNE

Abstract

AIM: To describe the historical events surrounding the development of the National League for Nursing (NLN) Academic Nurse Educator Certification Program (ANECP) and document its transition from a committee to a commission. **BACKGROUND:** During the latter half of the 20th century, certification became a demonstrated standard of excellence in nursing. A few visionaries suggested that nursing education itself was a specialty, but the timing for certification was not right. **METHOD:** The events have been studied through three primary sources: archived minutes, oral interviews, and the authors' eyewitness accounts. **RESULTS:** Growing pains, personnel changes, and the rapid growth from committee to commission occurred during a few short years. While the NLN made sound decisions during the change process by seeking evidence and the guidance of experts and consultants, unexpected challenges occurred. **CONCLUSION:**

The tremendous growth of the ANECP in its first years demonstrated that change was clearly desired so long as it was anchored in an evidence-based process focused on quality. [**Nursing Education Perspectives**, 34(5), 298–302, September/October 2013]

Preliminary Psychometric Analysis of the Modified Perceived Value of Certification Tool for the Nurse Educator

Tammy Barbé, PhD, RN, CNE

Abstract

AIM: The purpose of this study was to examine psychometric properties of the Perceived Value of Certification Tool© with a focus on nurse educator certification (PVCT-NE) in a sample of nurse educators. **BACKGROUND:** Greater understanding of faculty perceptions of certification is necessary to facilitate a strong cadre of nursing faculty, but research around nurse educator certification is limited by a lack of reliable and valid instruments to measure such perceptions. **METHOD:** Twenty-four nursing faculty from one university participated in the psychometric study, which involved completion of the PVCT-NE in a web-based survey format. **RESULTS:** Internal consistency reliability was excellent. Cronbach's alpha for the total PVCT-NE was .94 (.93 for the intrinsic subscale and .86 for the extrinsic subscale). A content validity index of .95 was obtained. **CONCLUSION:** There is preliminary evidence that the PVCT-NE is a reliable and valid instrument to measure perceived value of certification in nurse educators. [**Nursing Education Perspectives**, 36(4), 244–248, July/August 2015]

Candidates' First-Time Performance on the Certified Nurse Educator Examination

Tracy A. Ortelli, PhD, RN, CNE, ANEF

Abstract

AIM: This quantitative study examined the first-time pass/fail performance of 2,673 academic nurse educators who took the Certified Nurse Educator (CNE) examination between September 28, 2005 and September 30, 2011. **BACKGROUND:** This is the first research study designed to analyze candidates' first-time pass/fail performance on the CNE examination. **METHOD:** Descriptive statistics, chi-square test of independence, Pearson's r statistic, and binary logistic regression were performed. **RESULTS:** The chi-square test of independence revealed the lack of a statistically significant relationship between study participants' eligibility option and first-time pass/fail performance. Binary logistic regression revealed that a one-year increase in full-time experience resulted in a 1.05 times greater likelihood of passing the CNE examination (OR = 1.05; 95 percent CI 1.03, 1.06; $p = .00$). **CONCLUSION:** This study verifies the need for faculty development and mentoring for nurse educators with less than five years of full-time experience and supports recommendations for doctoral preparation. [**Nursing Education Perspectives**, 37(4), 189–193, July/August 2016]

CNE Certification Drive and Exam Results

Michelle M. Byrne, PhD, RN, CNOR, CNE; and Susan Welch, EdD, RN, CCRN, CNE

Abstract

The Certified Nurse Educator (CNE) is the only credential recognizing the advanced practice role of the academic nurse educator. This article provides information regarding a CNE Certification Drive for faculty in one school of nursing. Descriptive findings include pass rates and content-specific averages. An analysis of the relationship between the variables is offered for role (faculty vs. recent graduate), years of teaching, and differences in test scores. Results indicate no significant relationship between role and test results, $\chi2(1) = 1.11$, $p = .29$, and between years of teaching for those who passed ($M = 10.38$, $SD = 9.81$) versus those who failed ($M = 4.75$, $SD = 6.36$, $t(18) = 1.56$, $p = .14$). Additional research is needed to provide further understanding of variables linked with the CNE exam in multiple schools of nursing. [**Nursing Education Perspectives**, 37(4), 221–223, July/August 2016]

What Is the Value of Nurse Educator Certification? A Comparison Study of Certified and Noncertified Nurse Educators

Tammy Barbé, PhD, RN, CNE; and Laura P. Kimble, PhD, RN, FNP-C, FAHA, FAAN

Abstract

AIM: The purpose of this study was to examine differences in how certified nurse educators and noncertified nurse educators valued nurse educator certification. **BACKGROUND:** No studies have investigated the differences in perceptions of certified and noncertified nurse educators. Understanding these differences may influence how the nursing profession recognizes and promotes excellence within the academic nursing specialty. **METHOD:** Perceived Value of Certification Tool-Nurse Educator and demographic survey were administered via a web-based survey to a national sample of nursing faculty. **RESULTS:** Certified nurse educators valued certification with greater agreement than noncertified nurse educators. Personal accomplishment, personal satisfaction, and validation of knowledge were identified as the greatest rewards of certification. **CONCLUSION:** Nurse educators identified with intrinsic rewards of certification. Despite overall positive perceptions of nurse educator certification, strategies focused on extrinsic rewards may be necessary to increase certification rates. Such strategies may help overcome factors preventing educators from attaining certification. [**Nursing Education Perspectives**, 39(2), 66–71, March/April 2018]

Analysis of First-Time Unsuccessful Attempts on the Certified Nurse Educator Examination

John D. Lundeen, EdD, RN, CNE, COI

Abstract

AIM: This retrospective analysis examined first-time unsuccessful attempts on the Certified Nurse Educator (CNE) examination from September 2005 through September 2011 ($n = 390$). **BACKGROUND:** There are few studies examining certification within the academic nurse educator role. There is also a lack of evidence to assist nurse educators in understanding those factors that best support success on the CNE exam. **METHOD:** Nonexperimental, descriptive, retrospective correlational design using chi-square test of independence and factorial analyses of variance. **RESULTS:** A statistically significant relationship was found between first-time failure and highest degree obtained and institutional affiliation on the CNE exam. There was no statistically significant effect on mean scores in any of the six content areas measured by the CNE exam as related to highest degree or institutional affiliation. **CONCLUSION:** The findings from this study support a previous recommendation for faculty development, experience in the role, and doctoral preparation prior to seeking certification. [**Nursing Education Perspectives**, 39(2), 72–79, March/April 2018]

A Factor Analysis of the Perceived Value of Certification Tool for Nurse Educators: Evidence for Construct Validity

Tammy Barbé, PhD, RN, CNE; and Laura P. Kimble, PhD, RN, FNP-C, FAHA, FAAN

Abstract

AIM: The purpose of this study was to examine construct validity of the Perceived Value of Certification Tool for Nurse Educators (PVCT-NE). **BACKGROUND:** Preliminary testing of the PVCT-NE demonstrated content validity and strong evidence of internal consistency reliability. Construct validity evidence for the tool is lacking. **METHOD:** Using data from a descriptive study about nurses' perceived value of nurse educator certification, exploratory factor analysis was used to examine whether the factor structure of the PVCT-NE was consistent with the two-factor structure reported for the original PVCT. **RESULTS:** Data ($n = 221$) were analyzed using principal components analysis to identify factors. The observed two-factor solution and individual item loadings in this sample were consistent with the original PVCT's intrinsic and extrinsic value subscales and accounted for 64 percent of the total instrument variance. **CONCLUSION:** Overall, the PVCT-NE is a valid tool to measure perceived value of certification in nurse educators. [**Nursing Education Perspectives**, 39(3), E2–E6, May/June 2018]

PRESIDENT'S MESSAGE

Certification for Nurse Educators: A Mark of Excellence Celebrating 10 Years

Marsha Howell Adams, NLN President 2013–2015

[**Nursing Education Perspectives**, 36(4), 207, July/August 2015]

Throughout my time as president of the National League for Nursing and before, I spoke and wrote about the importance of excellence in nursing education. Excellence means not settling for the status quo. It always involves striving to be the best one can be.

One respected illustration of excellence for nurse faculty is the designation certified nurse educator (CNE®). Nurse educators who proudly include CNE in their credentials are recognized for their dedication to and investment in nursing education and nursing, and for their professional accomplishments and commitment to attaining the nurse educator competencies.

In 2005, the NLN published "Transforming Nursing Education," which recommends that "faculty identify themselves as advanced practice nurses since teaching is an advanced practice role that requires specialized knowledge and advanced education and since certification now exists as a way to recognize expertise in the role" (www.nln.org/about/position-statements/archived-position-statements, italics added). The Certified Nurse Educator Program, now 10 years old, first received national accreditation in 2009 from the National Commission for Certifying Agencies, renewed in 2014.

The mission of the NLN's Nurse Educator Certification Program is to promote excellence in the advanced specialty role of the academic nurse educator. The goals are to acknowledge the certified nurse educator as an advanced specialty role; recognize the role's knowledge, skills, and abilities required to demonstrate excellence; reinforce the nurse educator competencies; and promote lifelong learning through professional development. As of May 31, 2015, we have 4,887 individuals who have earned the CNE designation. What an accomplishment!

Eligibility requirements for taking the CNE exam have evolved over time and are based on the results of multiple CNE practice analyses. A practice analysis assesses activities undertaken when implementing roles and responsibilities required for a particular professional role. Presently, there are two options whereby an individual can sit for the certification exam. The individual must hold an active RN license and have either: a) a master's, post-master's, or doctoral degree with emphasis in nursing education or graduate-level education courses (nine hours), or b) a master's or doctoral degree in nursing, other than nursing education, and two years of experience in an academic nursing program within the last five years.

I recommend that you visit the NLN website for detailed information about fees and registration (www.nln.org/professional-development-programs/Certification-for-Nurse-Educators). For those of you who already hold the CNE designation, the website offers information about recertification. On the website is a link to the Certified Nurse Educator (CNE) Handbook, which contains invaluable information and resources to promote success on the exam.

I received my initial CNE designation in 2007 and was recertified in 2012. I found the practice exam to be a huge asset in preparing for the exam because it helped identify gaps in my knowledge and allowed me to focus my preparation time on certain areas. One can also choose to take a live NLN-sponsored review course, given throughout the country on a regular basis and as a preconference option at the NLN Education Summit. In addition, Dr. Linda Caputi has edited the NLN's Certified Nurse Educator Review, available for purchase from the NLN Bookstore (nln.lww.com), an essential text for aspiring CNEs and nurse educators across the academic spectrum.

The CNE designation sends a message to our students and our profession about how we value nursing education. I am very proud of my certification as an academic nurse educator and strongly encourage you to join me. In fact, each year at the NLN Education Summit, I, like my peers, carry a handsome red canvas bag signifying that I am a CNE. At the Summit in 2014, red honor cords were introduced for nurse educators to wear during graduation ceremonies. They were a hit.

At the 2015 NLN Education Summit, "A New World of Innovation and Technology," we will hold a special celebration for CNEs to recognize the 10th anniversary of the program. The NLN and its membership are doing great things. I hope you will be there and help us celebrate.

QUICK READS AND HEADLINES FROM THE NLN

Preparing for Certification in Nursing Education

Teresa Shellenbarger, DNSc, RN, CNE, ANEF

[**Nursing Education Perspectives**, 29(6), 330–332, November/December 2008]

Certification in nursing dates back to 1946 for nurse anesthetists (1). Now there are more than 65 certifying organizations, 95 different credentials, and certification in more than 130 nursing specialties (2). Nursing education joined the list of specialties that provide evidence of expertise through certification in fall 2006 with the administration of the first Certified Nurse Educator exam at the NLN Education Summit.

I recently completed the CNE exam and thought it might be helpful to share my experiences. I had been teaching nursing for more than 15 years when I made the decision to pursue certification. I saw certification as potentially helpful with faculty evaluation activities, such as tenure and promotion. Also, since I teach graduate nursing education courses, I hoped to gain some insight into the exam and become a role model for my students. It was particularly important to me to become certified before my students did.

Registering for the Exam

Having graduated before computer-adaptive NCLEX testing, I decided to take the computerized version of the certification exam, hoping that this experience would help me help my undergraduate students prepare for the NCLEX-RN. While pencil-and-paper testing was available when I registered, it is no longer an option. However, there are a variety of factors to consider when preparing to register for the exam.

First, it is essential to read the *CNE Candidate Handbook* and familiarize yourself with the eligibility requirements, policies and procedures, and fees. (All information and resources pertinent to the NLN Faculty Certification Program are online at www.nln.org/facultycertification/index.htm.) The application takes approximately 10 to 15 minutes to complete. You cannot schedule an examination test date and time until you have completed the registration process and have received a confirmation notice of eligibility.

Once your registration has been processed, you will receive directions for scheduling the exam date and time during a three-month testing window. Consider the timing of the exam and select a convenient date. You will also need to select the test site—one of 120 Applied Measurement Professionals testing centers located throughout the country.

Preparing for the Exam

The CNE exam was developed based on a practice analysis of nurse educators. This study yielded 119 tasks derived from the *Core Competencies of Nurse Educators with Task Statements* (3). These form the test blueprint, which is available online.

It is important to engage in self-reflection to identify areas of knowledge and any deficits you may have. *The CNE Candidate Handbook* offers sample questions, and a

65-item Self-Assessment Examination that follows the test map and format is available. This exam gives you the correct answers to questions, along with rationales, and provides for simulation of a computerized exam.

During my personal review, I identified that I had limited experience with online teaching and learning, diverse learners, and psychometrics for multiple-choice exams. Therefore, I focused on this content while reviewing other general areas.

The NLN provides a suggested reference list that may be helpful to review. Many of these classic nursing education sources, used in most graduate nursing education programs, provide the basis for the rationales for the responses. As part of the test preparation, you should also review *The Scope of Practice for Academic Nurse Educators* (4) and consider taking a formal review course. The NLN's biweekly *Faculty Development Bulletin* provides information about certification preparation courses offered throughout the country, and this information is available online at www.nln.org/facultydevelopment/workshopsandconf.htm.

Some faculty find it helpful to work with colleagues to prepare for the exam. Study groups or review sessions with other candidates who are preparing for the test may also be beneficial (5).

Test-Taking Reminders

As you prepare for the exam, keep good test-taking skills in mind. Remember that the people writing the test items are expert nurse educators who know test construction, and all items have been reviewed for content and structure. You will need to rely on your expert knowledge to be successful.

While studying, think prioritization of actions: What do you do first? What is the best response or action? What is the priority? Then, as you take the test, read the entire question, determine what is being asked, read and consider all answers completely, and then select the best response. Sometimes the response or action that you might use in a real situation is not a choice, so pick the best option from those available.

The Day of the Test

Use a variety of strategies that will help reduce your stress and allow you to arrive early for the exam. If you are traveling to an unfamiliar test site, be sure to have clear directions and a phone number for the test site. You may want to do a preliminary drive to be sure you know where to go and where to park.

Follow the instructions for what you are permitted to bring to the test site, typically two forms of identification and a wallet. Backpacks, bags, and purses are not allowed in the testing area. The exam takes three hours, and there are procedures you need to follow if you must exit for a break, so familiarize yourself with these rules. Wear comfortable clothes, preferably layers that can be removed if necessary.

During the testing session, you will need to complete a series of activities as part of the testing protocol. After providing identification, you will be shown to the testing area where you will complete a practice exam so that you will know how to proceed through the computer screens. You will be given scratch paper that must be returned at the end of the testing period. During my exam I did not have a lot of room to write. My testing space was an office cubicle with a traditional computer monitor and keyboard, which I needed to move aside to write my notes.

Make sure to monitor your time and track questions that you want to review. Since you are not penalized for incorrect answers, be sure to complete all questions. Although certain questions are considered experimental and will not count in the final grade, you will not know which these are.

A proctor was not present in the testing room when I took my exam, but all test takers were monitored by video camera. At the start of the exam, the computer was used to take my picture, which remained on the screen during the exam and was printed with the score report.

There are a number of other potential distractions. For example, exams of various lengths are given on the same day, so do not be alarmed if others leave early. When I took the nursing certification exam, I was the only person taking it. And I was seated next to a very nervous young man, retaking a failed exam, who continuously jiggled his leg up and down. It was a challenge to focus on my computer screen.

After you complete the exam you will need to complete a brief survey about the testing experience. After that is finished you will submit your scratch paper to the proctor. Unless a new exam is being piloted, you will receive your results immediately. The paper you receive will provide the dates of certification and list specific pass rates for the various sections of the test.

If you are unsuccessful on the exam, you will receive a detailed report of your performance. Take some time after the testing session to reflect upon your performance and consider strategies for remediation and retesting. Hopefully, with adequate preparation, you will be successful and will have a reason to celebrate as you join the growing number of CNE professionals.

Certification is good for five years. To renew, you can either take the test again or document professional development activities that relate to at least three competency areas. You will need to keep records of the activity, the date, and outcome and complete the certification renewal forms. Select applicants will need to submit supporting documentation as part of the recertification process.

References

1. Gaberson, K. B., Schroeter, K., Killen, A. R., & Valentine, W. A. (2003). The perceived value of certification by certified perioperative nurses. *Nursing Outlook, 51*(6), 272–276.

2. Briggs, L. A., Brown, H., Kesten, K., & Heath, J. (2006). Certification: A benchmark for critical care nursing excellence. *Critical Care Nurse, 26*(6), 47–53.

3. Ortelli, T. A. (2006). Defining the professional responsibilities of academic nurse educators: The results of a national practice analysis. *Nursing Education Perspectives, 27*(5), 242–246.

4. National League for Nursing. (2005). *The scope of practice for academic nurse educators*. New York, NY: Author.

5. Kohtz, C., Ferguson, P., Sisk, R., Gowda, C., Smith, J., & Fortson, A. (2008). The certified nurse educator exam: A plan for success [Quick Reads]. *Nursing Education Perspectives, 29*(1), 8–9.

Characteristics of Candidates Who Have Taken the Certified Nurse Educator (CNE) Examination: A Two-Year Review

Tracy Ortelli, MS, RN, CNE

[**Nursing Education Perspectives**, 29(2), 120–121, March/April 2008]

The National League for Nursing's Certified Nurse Educator (CNE) credential is the only professional credential that recognizes excellence in the advanced specialty role of the academic nurse educator. The CNE examination was initially offered in September 2005 to 206 qualified faculty representing 45 states and the District of Columbia. In the two years in which it has been available, 917 candidates have taken the examination, yielding 773 certified nurse educators. Educators with the CNE credential now represent all 50 states and the District of Columbia.

Eligibility Criteria

The CNE credential requires full-time faculty experience and a master's or doctoral degree in nursing. The two pathways that exist for eligibility are based on educational preparation and faculty experience.

To meet the criteria for Option A, nurse educators must have two years or more of full-time employment in the academic faculty role within the past five years. Further, they must possess a master's or doctoral degree in nursing with either a major emphasis in nursing education or nine or more credit hours of graduate-level education courses.

Nurse educators who possess a master's or doctoral degree in nursing with a major emphasis in a role other than nursing education are eligible for Option B if they have four or more years of full-time employment in the academic faculty role within the past five years. Of the CNE candidates, 64.8 percent met Option A criteria, and 35.2 percent met Option B criteria.

Demographic Data

Highest Degree Earned. The highest degree earned by the 917 candidates had nearly even distribution: 34.3 percent of candidates reported holding doctoral degrees; 34.4 percent held master's degrees in nursing with an education focus; and 31.3 percent held master's degrees in nursing with a focus other than nursing education.

To determine if the 917 candidates who took the CNE examination during this two-year period were representative of full-time nurse educators who teach in the United States, demographic data were compared to data described in *Nurse Educators 2006: A Report of the Faculty Census Survey of RN and Graduate Programs* (1). That report notes that nurse educators with doctoral degrees constitute 25.4 percent of the nation's faculty, and those with master's degrees constitute 68.9 percent of faculty. For CNE candidates, the percentages were comparable: 34.3 percent hold doctorates, and 65.7 percent hold master's degrees.

Primary Teaching Area. The Certified Nurse Educator examination is available to eligible candidates who teach in all levels of nursing education: practical, diploma, associate degree, baccalaureate, master's, and doctoral nursing programs. Of the candidates who took the CNE examination, 4.5 percent indicated that they taught primarily in practical nursing programs and 8.8 percent taught in diploma programs. The largest group taught in associate degree programs (39.1 percent), while 36.5 percent taught in baccalaureate programs and 11.0 percent taught primarily at the master's or doctoral level. It is interesting to note that while those who teach primarily in diploma programs represent 3.9 percent of the nation's faculty, they constitute 8.8 percent of the CNE candidate population.

Years of Full-Time Experience. The minimum number of years of full-time experience that a CNE candidate may have is two (within the past five years), provided the candidate possesses a master's or doctoral degree in nursing with an education focus. Of those who took the CNE examination, 23.4 percent indicated having two to five years of full-time experience; 39.5 percent reported 6 to 15 years; 25.3 percent reported 16 to 25 years; and 11.8 percent reported more than 26 years of full-time experience.

Rank. Nurse educators who hold the rank of instructor constitute the greatest percentage of CNE candidates (29.7 percent) followed by assistant professors (22.8 percent), associate professors (22.1 percent), and professors (16.6 percent). Of the CNE candidates, 9.1 percent indicated they did not hold a rank or title; those who did not indicate rank were typically employed in practical or diploma nursing programs.

Projected Retirement. Of the candidates who took the CNE examination during this reporting period, 14.9 percent indicated that they plan to retire within the next five years. Of great concern is the fact that nearly half (46.2 percent) reported that they plan to retire within the next decade and nearly three quarters (71.7 percent) within 15 years.

Overall Pass Rate

The cumulative pass rate for those who took the CNE examination between September 28, 2005 (pilot examination) and September 28, 2007 is 84.1 percent. The consistency of the pass rate over the past two years, during which time it was administered to more than 900 candidates, is one indication of the reliability of the CNE examination.

Summary and Future Research

The Certified Nurse Educator (CNE) examination is offered to a diverse group of qualified, full-time, academic nurse educators who represent the spectrum of nursing program types, academic ranks, years of experience, and educational preparation. Demographic data of CNE candidates reveal that interest in the Certified Nurse Educator credential is expressed by nurse educators in all career stages, who teach in all program types. The highest degree earned by candidates was evenly distributed and comparable to national faculty census data.

Candidates were most likely (39.4 percent) to report having six to 15 years of experience. The largest group of CNE candidates held the rank of instructor (29.7 percent) followed by assistant professor (22.8 percent) and associate professor (22.1 percent). Interest in earning the CNE credential may be associated with professional goals of promotion and tenure. Additional research is needed to explore the impact of certification on career advancement as well as the perceived value of certification.

Analysis of candidate performance on each content area of the test blueprint is planned. It is anticipated that these data will provide important information about candidates' knowledge about the Core Competencies of Nurse Educators© (2) as well as the professional development needs of our nation's faculty. The CNE credential, which is the first professional credential designed specifically for nursing faculty, is certain to have a significant influence on nursing education both locally and nationally. The National League for Nursing will closely and carefully evaluate these effects and encourages nurse researchers to investigate this new phenomenon in nursing education.

References

1. National League for Nursing. (2006). *Nurse educators 2006: A report of the faculty census survey of RN and graduate programs*. New York, NY: Author.

2. National League for Nursing. (2005). *Core competencies of nurse educators with task statements* [Online]. Retrieved from www.nln.org/facultydevelopment/pdf/corecompetencies.pdf

The NLN's Certified Nurse Educator Examination (CNE) Program Has Surpassed 5,000 and Gone Global

Larry Simmons, PhD, RN, CNE, NEA-BC

[**Nursing Education Perspectives**, 38(2), 110, March/April 2017]

At the end of 2016, the NLN Academic Nurse Educator Certification (CNE) program is proud to announce that the NLN has certified more than 5,300 nurse educators. This academic nurse certification program, now celebrating its 11th year, establishes nursing education as a specialty area of practice and creates a means for faculty to demonstrate their expertise in this role.

Certification in any field is a mark of professionalism. For academic nurse educators, certification communicates to students, peers, and the academic and health care communities that the highest standards of excellence are being met. By becoming credentialed as a Certified Nurse Educator (CNE), nurse educators serve as leaders and role models in their institutions and throughout the professional nursing community.

The mission of the CNE program is to promote excellence in the advanced specialty role of the academic nurse educator. The goals of the program are as follows:

▶ To distinguish academic nursing education as a specialty area of practice and an advanced practice role within professional nursing;

> To recognize the academic nurse educator's specialized knowledge, skills, and abilities and excellence in practice;

> To strengthen the use of core competencies of nurse educator practice; and

> To contribute to nurse educators' professional development.

History

From the program's conception in 2002, when the NLN convened a task group to develop academic nurse educator competencies; to the first pilot examination, administered in 2005 at the NLN Education Summit in Baltimore; to the evolution of the CNE Commission, with a Board of Commissioners; to the first approval of certification by the National Commission for Certifying Agencies (NCCA), a division of the Institute for Credentialing Excellence, in 2008; the program has surpassed expectations for championing the vital role of the academic nurse educator. In 2013, recertification of the program resulted in another five years of NCCA approval.

An exciting recent development has been the opening of the CNE program to global testers. The NLN has affiliated with CGFNS International, Inc. (www.cgfns.org) for validation of eligibility credentials for potential candidates from the international community. As said by NLN president Dr. Anne Bavier, "This partnership has been borne out of long years of collaboration and the complementary strengths that each organization will bring to making the CNE credential available and accessible to nurse educators seeking this leadership recognition in their respective countries." To date, nurse educators in Estonia, the Bahamas, and Germany have successfully passed the CNE examination. Nurse faculty outside the US seeking certification must first apply to CGFNS to have their qualifications evaluated for eligibility. Once approved, faculty may apply to the NLN for authorization to take the CNE examination.

Developing a New Examination

In 2015, the NLN convened a task group to identify competencies for the role of the clinical nurse instructor. These competencies and related task statements were based on current evidence-based literature and developed by educators from both education and practice. In fall 2016, the competencies were presented to the NLN Board of Governors for consideration of creating a new certification examination for clinical nurse educators. The work has now been delegated to the CNE Commission and will proceed through 2017. An NLN publication is also being developed by members of the task group to provide a comprehensive summary of the competencies; it will be available prior to completion of the competency examination. Look for announcements of the examination with a current target date of 2018.

Summary

The NLN is proud and confident that the Academic Nurse Educator Certification program offers quality certification for nurse educators and will continue to meet its goal to advance nurse educator specialty practice. The CNE Board of Commissioners strives to maintain a quality program and pursue new opportunities to enhance the program in the future. More information about the program is available on the NLN website: http://www.nln.org/Certification-for-Nurse-Educators.

Development of the Certified Nurse Educator Certification Exam: A Spotlight on Competencies, Scoring, and Security

Larry Simmons, PhD, RN, CNE, NEA-BC, and Linda Christensen, EdD, JD, RN, CNE

[**Nursing Education Perspectives**, 39(3):196, May/June 2018]

To a nurse educator taking a certification exam, the experience may seem similar to that of a student taking an instructor-created exam, but the process is very different, particularly with regard to test development. As we are often asked about the development and scoring of the NLN Certified Nurse Educator certification exam, following is a brief explanation of how the exam was originally developed, how it remains relevant to current practice, how it is scored, and how security is assured.

Test Development

Certification exams are the end-product of a rigorous test development process. The genesis of certification begins with the identification of the subject matter content/practice competencies and accompanying task statements for the role, which are derived from current literature. The competencies and task statements become the basis for the development of a practice analysis survey by a panel of subject matter experts. Results of the practice analysis are used to develop a test blueprint that outlines and guides test development. To ensure that the test blueprint remains reflective of the current practice of the role, the practice analysis survey is repeated every four to six years.

Subject matter experts write specific test items, each linked to a competency and task statement of the test plan. In addition, each test item must be referenced to current practice literature and conform to the best practices of writing standardized test items. Once the items are developed, they are pilot tested so that the statistical data for the items can be collected and analyzed. Based on item analysis, the test item may be retained "as is" (making it an active exam item suitable for use as a scored item on a test), revised, or deleted. If the item is revised, it must again be piloted before it can be considered active.

Data-Driven Scoring

The NLN certification program uses a minimum of two forms of the certification exam at any one time. Each form must strictly conform to the test blueprint, but the actual test items will vary. Test development committees (TDCs), composed of subject matter experts, are integral in the exam process. The TDC reviews the statistical performance of the individual test items, as well as overall exam performance validity and reliability.

This process is data driven. No arbitrary decisions about test items are made during the development and review process.

The passing score for each exam form is set by a method called "cut score setting." The cut score refers to the number of questions that must be answered correctly to pass the exam. The TDC uses a variety of statistical processes in analyzing data to set the cut score, such as the Angoff method or a more general equating method. The final cut score is determined by the TDC in collaboration with experienced psychometricians.

Because there are two forms of the certification exam, each exam's statistics must be examined independently to determine its specific cut score. It is therefore possible that the two exams may have different scores required for passing, with the slightly more difficult exam having a slightly lower passing score.

Test development activities remain a highly secure process. Information about test items is not shared by anyone outside of the test development meetings. Access to the test bank for review is strictly limited to the TDC members and tightly controlled by the agency that provides test administration to candidates.

Periodically, a post-testing candidate requests a review of test items. This is never permitted with a certification exam, as these exams are high stakes testing for a profession. The security of exams must never be impugned.

Another occasional request is to discard one or more test items from a tester's exam based upon the rationale that there was more than one correct response. Certification items are written so that there is only one correct response that is easily referenced to current literature. Sometimes testers state that certain test items did not reflect their role as a nurse educator. It is important to remember that the certification test is based upon the role competencies and task statements for the role and not on individual practice.

One similarity between a nurse educator's taking a certification exam and a student taking an instructor-created classroom exam has to do with preparation. A well-prepared student for a classroom exam will know generally what type of content will be covered and will study accordingly. A well-prepared nurse educator will review the candidate handbook, identify the test plan, and prepare accordingly.

The Academic Clinical Nurse Educator

Linda Christensen, EdD, JD, RN, CNE, and Larry E. Simmons, PhD, RN, CNE, NEA-BC

[**Nursing Education Perspectives**, 40(3), 196, May/June 2019]

In the early 2000s, the National League for Nursing (NLN) identified the need to articulate the role of the academic nurse educator. This resulted in the identification of the full scope of the role of the academic nurse educator through the development of evidence-based competencies and related task statements. In early 2015, the idea for articulating the specific role of the academic clinical nurse educator began to take root.

The NLN formed a task group to analyze the literature with the idea of developing role competencies and task statements related to the academic clinical nurse educator role. The task group arrived at consensus on the role and presented the resulting competencies and related task statements to the NLN community for review and feedback. After comments were considered by the task group, the final version of the competencies and task statements was released (September, 2018).

Based on the delineation of the role of the academic clinical nurse educator, a decision was made to move forward with the development of a certification examination. A practice analysis was developed and academic clinical nurse educators were asked to assist in validation of the task statements associated with the role. The results of the practice analysis provided the basis for the creation of a certification test blueprint. After certification exam test items were developed, two forms of an exam were established, and pilot testing was conducted in the summer/fall of 2018. After passing scores were psychometrically set, the Certified Academic Clinical Nurse Educator (CNE©cl) certification program was officially launched in October 2018.

Definition of Practice

The academic clinical nurse educator may be known by a variety of titles (e.g., clinical faculty, part-time faculty, adjunct faculty, preceptor, clinical instructor). A core definition was developed that would encompass many of the titles being used and clearly delineate the professional role attributes. "The academic nurse educator facilitates the learning of nursing students throughout clinical components of an academic nursing program. The educator is guided…by the faculty of the nursing program and is accountable to the nursing program for providing fair evaluations of learners' performance in meeting expected learning outcomes" (NLN, 2019).

The academic clinical nurse educator submits evaluations of learners' performance that result in academic credit for the clinical learning experience. The academic clinical nurse educator also provides direct supervision of the student learner in the clinical setting. The purpose of the CNEcl certification exam is to validate expertise in the defined role of the academic clinical nurse educator. The goals of the CNEcl certification are as follows:

1. Distinguish academic clinical nursing education as a specialty area of practice.
2. Recognize the academic clinical nurse educator's specialized knowledge, skills, and abilities and excellence in clinical teaching.
3. Strengthen the use of selected core competencies of academic clinical nurse educator practice.
4. Contribute to academic clinical nurse educator clinical practice.

Final Thoughts

The mission of the NLN is to promote excellence in nursing education to build a strong and diverse nursing workforce to advance the health of our nation and the global community. Various products and services of the NLN, such as certification, contribute to meeting the mission. Since the earlier work that established the role of the academic nurse educator, those competencies and task statements have been used as a basis for faculty development, faculty evaluation, curriculum development, and research into the faculty role (Halstead, 2018). The articulation of the academic clinical nurse educator role has the same potential to promote nursing education overall.

Certification in any field stands as achieving a mark of excellence for the certificants. Certification, particularly in nursing education, is viewed as a mark of distinction and goal attainment for all nursing faculty striving to excel in educational and practice endeavors.

References

Halstead, J. A. (Ed.). (2018). *NLN core competencies for nurse educators: A decade of influence*. Washington, DC: National League for Nursing.

National League for Nursing. (2019). *Certified Academic Clinical Nurse Educator (CNE®cl): 2019 Candidate handbook*. Retrieved from www.nln.org/Certification-for-Nurse-Educators/cnecl/cne-cl-handbook

Shellenbarger, T. (Ed.). (2018). *Clinical nurse educator competencies: Creating an evidence-based practice for academic clinical nurse educators*. Washington, DC: National League for Nursing.

Acknowledgments

The NLN Core Competencies for Nurse Educators (2005) and the Clinical Nurse Educator Competencies (2019) were developed by nursing education leaders who had the vision to clearly articulate the advanced practice roles of the Academic Nurse Educator and the Academic Clinical Nurse Educator. Their work demonstrates the NLN mission to "promote excellence in nursing education to build a strong and diverse nursing workforce to advance the health of our nation and the global community" (NLN, 2019).

The Academic Nurse Educator Competencies were Developed by the NLN Task Group on Nurse Educator Competencies (2002–2004).

Judith A. Halstead, DNS, RN (Chair)

Wanda Bonnel, PhD, RN

Barbara Chamberlain, MSN, RN, CNS, C, CCRN

Pauline M. Green, PhD, RN

Karolyn R. Hanna, PhD, RN

Carol Heinrich, PhD, RN

Barbara Patterson, PhD, RN

Helen Speziale, EdD, RN

Elizabeth Stokes, EdD, RN

Jane Sumner, PhD, RN

Cesarina Thompson, PhD, RN

Diane M. Tomasic, EdD, RN

Patricia Young, PhD, RN

Mary Anne Rizzolo, EdD, RN, FAAN (NLN Staff Liaison)

The 2012 Revisions to the Scope of Practice publication were Developed by the NLN CNE 2012 Task Group.

Nancy Sharts-Hopko, PhD, RN, CNE, FAAN (CNE Commission Chair)

Marsha Adams, DNS, RN, CNE, ANEF

Pamela DiVito-Thomas, PhD, RN, CNE

Tara Hulsey, PhD, RN, CNE

Jan Nick, PhD, RN, CNE, ANEF

Judy K. Ogans, MS, RN, CNE

Linda S. Christensen, JD, MSN, RN (NLN Staff Liaison)

Ayana Nickerson (NLN Staff Liaison)

Larry E. Simmons, PhD, RN, NEA-BC, CNE (NLN Staff Liaison)

The Academic Clinical Nurse Educator Competencies were Developed by the NLN Task Group on Academic Clinical Nurse Educator Competencies (2015–2017).

Wanda Bonnel, PhD, APRN, ANEF

Melora D. Ferren, MSN, RN-BC

Erin Killingsworth, PhD, RN, CNE

John D. Lundeen, EdD, RN, CNE, COI

Amber M. Patrick, PhD, RN, CNE, COI

Teresa Shellenbarger, PhD, RN, CNE, ANEF

Linda S. Christensen, EdD, JD, RN, CNE (NLN Staff Liaison)

Larry E. Simmons, PhD, RN, NEA-BC, CNE (NLN Staff Liaison)